The Vaccines for Children Program

The Vaccines for Children Program

A Critique

Robert M. Goldberg

The AEI Press

Publisher for the American Enterprise Institute

WASHINGTON, D.C.

1995

This report was prepared under a grant from the Albert Sabin Vaccine Foundation. The author is grateful for the foundation's support. The opinions and conclusions herein contained are the author's alone. The author is also responsible for any errors or omissions.

ISBN 0-8447-7052-3

1 3 5 7 9 10 8 6 4 2

The AEI Press
Publisher for the American Enterprise Institute
1150 17th Street, N.W., Washington, D.C. 20036

Contents

The Vaccines for Children Program—A Critique

Robert M. Goldberg

The Vaccines for Children Program (VFC) was the Clinton administration's first shot in the battle to pass the Health Security Act. Envisioned as a symbol of President Clinton's commitment to social change, the program was designed to be a single-payer system for childhood vaccines, covering everyone up to the age of eighteen. Today, the program is in disarray. It is an entitlement of nearly $1 billion a year, and in the words of Senator Dale Bumpers, it "will not immunize one additional kid."

The real failure of VFC, however, has been the willingness of the Clinton administration and its allies to rewrite and distort the immunization "problem" to fit a more far-reaching political agenda. The administration claimed early on that the high cost of vaccines was causing babies to go unimmunized. Nothing is further from the truth. Immunization rates among children under two for each of the major antigens (polio, diphtheria-tetanus-pertussis [DTP], and measles-mumps-rubella [MMR]) are at or near 90 percent, the highest ever. Enough vaccine is already available to immunize at least 150 percent of all infants at little or no cost. Despite the fact that government studies show that children in the inner cities either have insurance coverage, access to free vaccines, or see a doctor eight to sixteen times in the first two years of life, low immunization rates still persist. And among that group of poor children, demonstration projects show that allowing parents simply to obtain a three-month (instead of a one-month) supply of Women, Infants, and Children (WIC) coupons if their children are immunized on time doubles immunization rates.

But VFC could not have been forged on the anvil of success. To secure its passage and status as an entitlement, the Clinton administration had to create a crisis in childhood immunizations. So it ignored the real roots of the immunization program, as well as the genuine progress that was being made. Even now that the truth about immunization coverage is becoming better known, program supporters in and out of the administration still cling to the contention that vaccine costs are driving down immunization rates. VFC was never meant to be a specific solution to a simple problem. Instead, it is a classic case of how easy it is to ignore social progress and manufacture a crisis to support the growth of entitlements.

Despite the administration's mishandling of the program—which included a plan to store nearly 40 percent of the nation's pediatric vaccine supply in a warehouse filled with paint solvents and paper clips—and despite the direct evidence that there is no immunization crisis, VFC is still growing. President Clinton mentions immunizations along with school lunches and education spending as items that should be spared by budget cutters. Indeed, the administration is going to great lengths to protect VFC from budget cuts.

If the program succeeds, it will ensure that by 1998 nearly $7 billion will have been spent to solve a problem that does not exist at the expense of other disease-prevention measures. Compared with other social and health-related problems, low immunization rates are a manageable concern. By continuing to preserve the program, the administration is ensuring that the government will persist in borrowing against our children's future and spending against their needs. How the nation arrived at this dismal state of affairs is the theme of this study.

A Brief History of Federal Vaccine Programs

Prior to the enactment of VFC, the federal government had a modest and advisory role in supporting local immunization programs. For the most part, federal assistance took the form of grants and technical assistance to help state and local public health agencies improve disease surveillance and promote disease prevention activities. Beginning with the Vaccine Assistance Act of 1962, the federal government provided rural areas with funding to immunize children not regularly receiving this care in the school program. The act lapsed in 1968, and the following year Congress cleared a bill opposed by the Nixon administration authorizing a two-year program of grants to the states for communicable-disease control and vaccinations.

In 1977, the secretary for Health, Education, and Welfare, Joseph Califano, launched an expanded federal effort to immunize children against polio, measles, mumps, rubella, whooping cough, diphtheria, and tetanus. At the time, Califano estimated that 65 percent of all children not receiving a full series of immunizations came from lower-income families. The program provided state and local health agencies with training, technical assistance, and money for vaccine purchases. Such funding was intended to supplement categorical and matching grant programs for comprehensive public health services.[1]

Since the Califano initiative, the heart of federal support for immunization efforts has been the authority of the government under Section 317 of the Public Health Act.

Known as "317," the program now consists of two components: federal purchase of vaccines for public health clinics, and a combination of grants and technical assistance to build up immunization and disease prevention activities at the state and local levels. In addition, immunization services are covered under Medicaid, Healthy Start, and Maternal and Child Health block grants.

Federal spending for immunization services increased steadily during the 1980s, and, under President Bush, federal purchases of vaccines nearly tripled, growing from $98.2 million in fiscal year 1988 to $297 million in fiscal year 1992. In addition, Bush added $46 million to improve immunization delivery to preschool children. Funding was provided to purchase more vaccines and to support the development of community Immunization Action Plans (IAP).

The Genesis of VFC

During the 1992 presidential election campaign, President and Mrs. Clinton asserted that the measles epidemic was the result of the Bush administration's failure to provide poor and middle-class children with access to vaccines. In calling for a program to create a children's vaccine entitlement, the campaign followed the lead of the Children's Defense Fund—of which Mrs. Clinton was once a board member—which issued a report blaming the cost of vaccines for creating a "lethal chain of events" that led to children's death from measles.

The campaign pledge to create a vaccines program for children was to become the first domestic policy initiative of the new administration. White House advisors saw the vaccine issue as an excellent way to position the president on health care and to demonstrate his willingness to take on special interests that might stand in the way. At a February 1993 appearance, President Clinton announced the new Vaccines for Children Program. In so doing, he lashed out at the shockingly high price of vaccines and asserted that it was unconscionable to place profits above the health of children.

The kickoff for VFC bore all the markings of a dress rehearsal for the health care reform program. Health and Human Services (HHS) Secretary Donna Shalala announced the creation of VFC surrounded by the bill's congressional sponsors—including the chairmen of congressional committees having jurisdiction over health, such as Senator Edward Kennedy, House Energy and Commerce Committee Chairman John Dingell, and the Health subcommittee chairman, Henry Waxman. Marian Wright Edelman was also on hand—the president of the Children's Defense Fund, the organization that developed the idea of childhood vaccine entitlement.

In her announcement on the new entitlement, Secretary Shalala said, "The Comprehensive Child Immunization Act of 1993 is a sound and cost-effective investment in America's future health and productivity. It will become a cornerstone in the administration's national health care reform plan—a plan that will emphasize prevention and provide all Americans with the security of knowing that their basic health care needs will be met."[2]

Using the Rhetoric of Crisis and Failure to Pass VFC

The campaign to secure passage of VFC was organized to establish the failure of the current immunization system and the impending immunization crisis. The central theme was that immunization rates are low because vaccine prices are too high, and, without a vaccine entitlement, too many of America's children would be exposed to the risk of disease.

The message came through clearly that rising vaccine prices were denying children essential health care. Every major newspaper reported, without question, that vaccine prices rose 800 percent and that immunization

5

rates were the lowest in a decade—lower than in most countries that have universal purchase. (Such reports ignored the fact that 64 percent of the cost of private-practice immunizations came from physician fees and that nearly two-thirds of the increase in vaccine cost was a result of new vaccines and a federal excise tax.) Hearings chaired by Senator Donald Riegle focused on the pricing practices of vaccine companies and alleged price differentials in vaccines sold here and abroad.

The theme of the hearing was how "pediatricians and family physicians routinely referred children in their offices who needed immunizations to public clinics because of high costs. The result is that children miss opportunities to be vaccinated and are left vulnerable to disease."[3] The cost of the complete series of vaccines—which rose from $11 in 1977 to about $200 in 1993, due to the addition of two new vaccines (for hepatitis B and haemophilus influenzae B) and a federal excise tax—was cited as the key reason why children were not being immunized properly.

Naturally, high vaccine prices were blamed for the failure of the United States to immunize its children fully. Indeed, the Children's Defense Fund rereleased information showing that the United States has lower immunization rates than most countries. According to that organization, the "United States ranks 70th in the world behind Burundi, Iran, Indonesia, Cuba, Jamaica, and Trinidad and Tobago, and U.S. preschool immunization rates, according to all available measures, declined during the 1980s."[4]

Secretary Shalala testified that the immunization rate for children under two was 55 percent, and "that the United States has one of the lowest immunization rates for preschool children when compared with European countries."[5] That figure was used as effective and stark evidence of the need for VFC and became an important reason for passage of the entitlement.

6

In an environment defined by crisis and guilt there was never any question about the accuracy of the administration's argument or a debate about the need for VFC. Even Democratic legislators who questioned the utility of VFC felt they could not directly confront a newly elected Democratic president on his first major domestic policy initiative, particularly one of such importance to both the president and Mrs. Clinton. In fact, such was the pressure from the administration to get VFC enacted that the money allocated to pay for the program was obtained by making cuts in Medicare.

As a result, congressional resistance came in the form of objections to the amount of money spent, not to the program's purpose. For the most part, opponents of universal purchase countered with a proposal that would have allowed states to purchase vaccine used in the Medicaid program with federal dollars only. With the exception of a bill introduced by Senator Dale Bumpers, a legislator with extensive experience in immunization issues, no measures were introduced that linked funding to improved vaccination rates. Statements from public health officials that lack of access to vaccines was not a problem were ignored.

Vaccine companies were also ambivalent about taking on the issue directly. While the industry wanted to defeat the measure outright, it never pursued such a strategy. Instead, each of the companies supported a measure introduced by Senator John Danforth that would have had the federal government purchasing vaccines for the Medicaid program in addition to the existing Centers for Disease Control (CDC) purchase. While companies complained that VFC would undermine future investment in new vaccines, they blunted their argument by participating in the program despite that view.

In its final form, VFC had all the elements of a single-payer health care system. Although the size of the initial appropriation was reduced and certain limits were placed on eligibility (no one with insurance that covered vaccines would receive free ones), the vaccine entitlement and the virtual elimination of a private market for vaccine purchase and delivery became law. Price controls were imposed on existing vaccines. New vaccine prices would have to be negotiated with the administration. Fee caps were imposed on pediatricians, and doctors were prohibited from charging a fee for free vaccines if parents said they could not afford it.

In addition, an unelected board of pediatricians was given the power to determine which new vaccines would be added to the entitlement. All children under the age of eighteen were eligible for free vaccines except for those whose insurance plans covered immunizations. Doctors were to inquire about insurance coverage but were not required to verify whether parents were providing accurate information. The government would centrally control the ordering, storage, shipping, and delivery of pediatric vaccines.[6] True, Congress had scaled back the scope of the program—prohibiting children with insurance plans covering immunizations from receiving VFC vaccines. But only in Washington is it deemed a "compromise" to save a program that was not needed in the first place.

Evaluating the Need for VFC

The effort to cloud the issue of immunization rates in the rhetoric of crisis has obscured the fact that before VFC's enactment, immunization rates in the United States were rising and reaching record levels. As Dr. Walter Orenstein, director of the Centers for Disease Control and Prevention's (CDCP) National Immunization Program, testified, "Immunization rates are the highest ever."[7] As figure 1 suggests, Secretary Shalala's contention that immunization rates were at 55 percent was inaccurate. In fact, Shalala was using 1986 data, while 1992 data were

FIGURE 1
VACCINATION RATES FOR CHILDREN AGED
TWO YEARS AND UNDER, 1992 AND 1994
(percent)

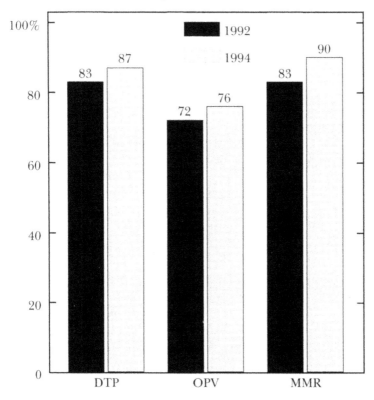

NOTE: DTP = diphtheria-tetanus-pertussis; OPV = oral polio vaccine;
MMR = measles-mumps-rubella.
SOURCE: Centers for Disease Control and Prevention.

available at HHS. The old data depicted an immunization "crisis," while the then-current statistics showed that
immunization rates for each major shot were near the
administration's 90 percent goal and rising. Shalala never
discussed the CDCP data showing immunization levels
for each of the three major sets of shots in 1992 for two-

year-olds at about 83 percent. Yet in other parts of her testimony she used the 1992 data to refer to the number of poor children not fully immunized—data that were not made publicly available until January 1994.[8]

At the time VFC was introduced, there was enough evidence that every child had access to vaccine at little or no cost, which prompted Dr. Orenstein to assert: "Anyone who is motivated can get immunized in this country today."[9] The table below, based on 1991 data obtained from the CDCP, affirms Dr. Orenstein's assessment. Figure 2 shows that the CDCP purchases between 71 percent and 88 percent of the vaccine necessary to immunize all two-year-olds.

This number needs some qualification. The CDCP has a policy of buying vaccines for a projected number of children who need to catch up on their immunization schedule. Therefore, some of the "317 program" vaccine purchase takes the catchup doses into account. But there is currently enough public-sector vaccine available to immunize nearly all children under the age of two.

Did Immunization Referrals Cause the Measles Epidemic?

As will be discussed later, supporters of VFC rest their case for the entitlement on the "evidence" that low immunization rates are the result of having pediatricians refer parents who cannot afford to pay for vaccines to public health clinics. Indeed, health researchers recently asserted that "such immunization referrals were first reported at the end of the last decade, when the cost of the basic series of childhood vaccines had risen sharply and the United States experienced a multi-year measles epidemic."[10] The implication, of course, is that the measles epidemic was caused by the high price of vaccines (see figure 3).

This line of argument is flatly contradicted by an overwhelming body of empirical evidence gathered in

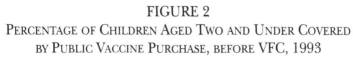

FIGURE 2

PERCENTAGE OF CHILDREN AGED TWO AND UNDER COVERED
BY PUBLIC VACCINE PURCHASE, BEFORE VFC, 1993

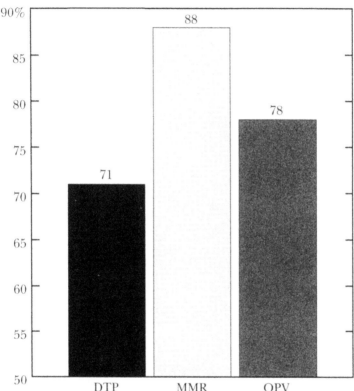

SOURCE: Centers for Disease Control and Prevention.

the wake of the measles epidemic. It is also contradicted by the fact that, prior to VFC, the measles epidemic was controlled without spending one additional dollar on vaccine coverage.

In fact, the containment of the measles epidemic is another success story, not a continuing crisis. After declining from an average of 600,000 cases of measles each year before the measles vaccine was introduced in

FIGURE 3
MEASLES IN PERSPECTIVE, 1960–1993
(number of cases)

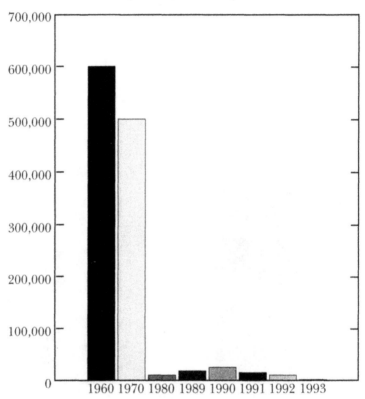

SOURCE: Centers for Disease Control and Prevention.

1972, measles cases fell dramatically and reached a low of about 1,500 cases in 1983. Between 1983 and 1988 the number of measles cases rose slightly but steadily. Measles cases rose sharply to 18,000 in 1989 and to 25,000 in 1990. By 1991, measles cases dropped off by 65 percent, and by 1993, only several hundred measles cases were reported.

The measles epidemic was confined to a handful of poor, largely minority neighborhoods. Nearly one-third of all cases were reported in three cities—Houston, Los Angeles, and Chicago—with the remainder occurring in Dallas, Milwaukee, and New York. On average, Hispanic and black preschool children in urban areas were seven to nine times more likely to contract measles as were non-white children. Ironically, "although immunization levels are 97 to 98 percent at the time of enrollment in school, they are reported to be as low as 50 percent among two-year-olds in some inner-city populations."[11]

What were the reasons for the measles epidemic in these neighborhoods? Lack of access to vaccines and social services was not at issue. First, an investigation of the measles epidemic found that "only two states reported inadequate vaccine supplies in the public sector for routine immunization of preschoolers, despite the prevalent belief that this was a major problem."[12] One of those states, it turned out, was Washington, which buys vaccine for all its children!

Second, the report went on to observe that "although inner-city preschool children are often described as hard to reach, many of these children are in regular contact with public assistance programs that typically see enrolled families every month. The failure to vaccinate adequately many children currently enrolled in public assistance programs suggests that many of the potential benefits gained by recent expansion in Medicaid eligibility to a much larger group of poor and near-poor preschoolers may not be realized unless steps are taken to ensure that immunization is an integral part of program activities."[13]

Hence, the measles epidemic had little to do with vaccine prices or overcrowded public health clinics. Instead, missed opportunities to vaccinate—that is, times when infants were actually in the doctor's office but never received a measles shot—were the cause of the outbreak. To the extent that children had several chances to receive a measles shot but did not do so at all or in a timely fashion, the question of why this happened becomes paramount.

Several studies sponsored by the Centers for Disease Control and Prevention found that low immunization rates, where they existed, had little to do with the reasons given by VFC proponents and repeated by the media. These studies, the most carefully conducted and controlled research of its kind, looked at immunization patterns in Chicago, Philadelphia, Los Angeles, and Baltimore. While such reports found that poor black children were less likely to be immunized than children from other races or income groups, poverty or lack of access to free vaccines had nothing to do with low immunization rates.

What the studies found was a complex set of behavioral factors that have little to do with the benefits that entitlements like VFC provide. An excellent study was conducted by Bernard Guyer, et al., on immunization coverage and its relationship to preventive health care among poor children in Baltimore. Dr. Guyer's study is important for its comprehensiveness and thoroughness, and his conclusions are strikingly similar to those found in studies conducted in Philadelphia and Los Angeles. Dr. Guyer's study found that:

> The low immunization coverage levels observed in Baltimore exist despite the presence of a large network of primary health care facilities to which these children have access and despite the availability of health insurance (via Medicaid), sufficient preventive health visits during the first two years of life, and free vaccine.[14]

More important to solving the problem that exists, the study found that infants who received their first DTP shot on time (within three months of birth) were three times as "likely to receive their third DTP shot on time and twice as likely to be up-to-date at twenty-four months than the infants who were delayed in receiving the first shot of DTP."

In probing further, Dr. Guyer and his research team found that a combination of parental delay in seeking preventive care and provider practices at sick and well visits "serves to defer and delay achievement of age-appropriate immunization."[15]

Hence, the major reasons for the lack of complete and timely immunizations have largely to do with the initiation and sequencing of primary health care. Getting the first shot on time is an important factor regardless of the race, income, or insurance status of the parents. The later the first shot is administered, the more difficult it is to catch up and stay on schedule.

Dr. Guyer's findings, which are consistent with those derived from studies conducted in Philadelphia and Los Angeles, therefore suggest that cost or vaccine access is irrelevant to raising immunization rates where low rates exist.[16] Moreover, the study also indicates that simply leveraging from the first DTP shot may be an effective way to improve immunization rates.

From the outset, the real reasons for the measles epidemic and the nation's success in quickly controlling it were ignored. Instead, the measles epidemic was portrayed as a problem of poverty and thus inequality. It was used to demonstrate that an entitlement was needed to avoid a crisis. For example, the Children's Defense Fund blamed high vaccine prices for setting off what they termed the "lethal chain of events" that led to the epidemic.[17] From their perspective, high vaccine prices led to crowding in (or being turned away from) overburdened public health clinics, which in turn led to a decline in immunization rates, which of course led to the measles epidemic.

This rhetoric of guilt and failure also shaped the recommendations of the National Vaccine Advisory Committee (NVAC). The policy conclusions drawn by the NVAC have little bearing on the circumstances surrounding the measles epidemic that the committee itself reported, ignoring its own observations. For example, while it found that parents had adequate contact with Medicaid and other social services, the NVAC concluded that low immunization rates reflect, in part, "inadequate access to health care." Though it found no shortage of free vaccines except in two isolated situations, it asserted that "the high costs of vaccines...are often passed on to parents," who in turn are forced to seek immunization in already overtaxed public clinics.[18] Nor did the study explain why such circumstances were "barriers" to immunization when a child is not yet two, but are not obstacles at all when the child is five and needs the shots to get into school.

Raising Immunization Rates in Low-Income Areas without VFC

Indeed, the fact that parents are able to get their children fully immunized by age five suggests that some modest, low-cost intervention could raise immunization rates among the children under two, in areas where the problem persists. The key to raising vaccination levels would be to encourage parents and physicians to stay on schedule with all required shots. There is growing evidence that policies that reward such behavior can achieve dramatic results.

For example, the CDCP-sponsored experiments that link the receipt of Women, Infants, and Children (WIC) food coupons with getting children immunized on time have proved to be highly successful. Demonstration projects conducted in Dallas and Chicago screened parents for their children's immunization status. If the children were up to date, the parents could get a three-month supply of WIC coupons. If not, parents would have to return

FIGURE 4
THE EFFECT OF TYING ENTITLEMENTS TO IMMUNIZATION,
CHICAGO, 1994
(percent)

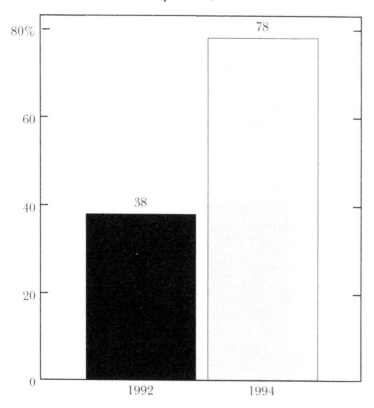

SOURCES: Women, Infants, and Children coupon project demonstration in Chicago, 1994; Centers for Disease Control and Prevention.

monthly to obtain WIC coupons until the children met the immunization schedule. The linkage had a dramatic effect on raising vaccination rates. The demonstration projects show that the voucher incentive is more effective than simply referring parents to a nurse or clinic after screening (see figures 4 and 5).

17

FIGURE 5
THE EFFECT OF TYING ENTITLEMENTS TO IMMUNIZATION, DALLAS, 1994
(percent)

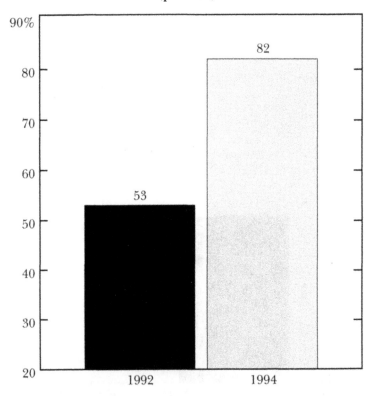

SOURCES: Women, Infants, and Children coupon project demonstration in Dallas, 1994; Centers for Disease Control and Prevention.

Similarly, Mississippi, a state with one of the lowest per capita incomes in the nation, and one with limited public resources to address the prevention of disease, has achieved one of the highest immunization levels for its two-year-old children of any state. According to Dr. F.E. Thompson, the state's health officer, "We have not found the availability of vaccine, or its cost, to be a significant barrier....The real barriers are our failure to remind parents of needed doses and our missed opportunities to immunize children [whom] we are already seeing."[19] By setting up a tracking and reminder system in its public clinics, many public health districts were able to raise completion levels of all two-year-olds to 90 percent without doing anything about the cost of vaccine.

Georgia has been able to double the immunization rates among its poor families without additional vaccine distribution. The point is that the VFC delivery system is not a solution to the problem of low immunization rates. Indeed, as Dr. Orenstein acknowledged in testimony last year, many clinics in Georgia have seen "without a major increase in funding, increased immunization levels among their clinic attenders from less than 40 percent to almost 80 percent."[20]

Hence, if immunization policies are based on existing empirical evidence and build on past success, it is possible to improve immunization rates in areas where it has traditionally been difficult to raise them. American children are more protected from disease now than ever before: for at least the past decade, enough free vaccine has been available to immunize each generation of newborns more than once. Immunization levels are nearly 100 percent at the time of enrollment in school. The measles epidemic was quickly controlled, and low cost immunization programs have been effective in immunizing hard-to-reach children. It is logically impossible that we could achieve all this success and simultaneously have some of the lowest immunization rates in the world. The numbers, largely ignored in the creation of VFC, prove it.[21]

Defense of the VFC—The "Crisis" of Immunization Referrals

Even though the increase in immunization rates took place before enactment and implementation of VFC, and in its original testimony the administration claimed vaccination rates were below 60 percent, the same administration is now taking credit for the record high immunization levels. In a section entitled "Preventing Disease through Immunization," the president's budget for fiscal 1996 proudly claims that it "has made substantial progress toward the goal of immunizing 90 percent of children up to age two by 1996. Immunization rates for some vaccines—such as three doses of DTP—almost reached that level by the end of 1993." The fact that VFC did not actually go into effect until October 1, 1994, and has hardly shipped any vaccine is ignored in this statement.

While the White House is proudly claiming progress, its allies and the CDCP are still insisting that immunization rates are low because parents cannot afford vaccines and because their doctors are referring them to public health clinics, which in turn "contribute significantly to lagging U.S. immunization rates."[22] This argument has a certain self-justifying logic to it, as long as one ignores the high immunization rates, the reasons for low rates in urban areas, and the success in raising rates among the poor. The evidence used to support this contention consists of surveys that ask physicians about their referral rates and of the assertion, largely unsupported by data, that states with universal vaccine-purchase programs have higher immunization rates than those without them.

The physician surveys do not answer the most important question: What happens to the children after they are told to go to a public health clinic? Dr. Orenstein, a leading researcher on the factors contributing to immunization rates, has stated, "There is no empirical evidence that physician referrals have any impact on immunization rates. There are so many variables that it is impossible to make any clear connection."[23]

Moreover, the surveys are deeply flawed. A widely touted study of referrals in New York asks doctors to recall whether they referred any patients to clinics over the past ten years and the reasons for the referral. The study is therefore flawed because doctors fail to follow a group of children from the referral to the clinic.

Finally, these surveys ignore three important facts. First, immunization rates have been *rising* since 1989, before the passage of VFC and after the addition of vaccines for haemophilus influenza B (HiB) and hepatitis B. Second, the same children facing a "referral crisis" manage to get their shots by age five. Indeed, CDC studies show that 98 percent of five-year-old children are fully immunized. Their two-year-old siblings and counterparts, in the same communities, the same families, and with access to the same free vaccines and health care, are not. And last, children who are required to be immunized before enrolling in day care and Head Start programs are also fully immunized. Intent on inventing a referral crisis, the Clinton administration and its supporters ignore the bottom line: that rates were rising before VFC, and that children are fully immunized when receipt of welfare benefits is tied to timely vaccination.

Ultimately, what will secure VFC's future is the desire of states to buy up vaccine at the federally controlled price. States have already counted the "savings" provided by VFC vaccine purchase and discount opportunities. Further, many governors see free vaccine as a quick way to provide voters with a benefit without having to pay for it directly. As a result, nearly thirty states want to buy up vaccines for all children, because VFC now requires that companies sell additional vaccine to states at the federally controlled price. The stiffest resistance to repealing VFC will likely come from states that want to buy more vaccine. Political self-interest alone, rather than the specific problem of low immunization rates for which free vaccine is not a solution, will be the factor deciding whether the program lives or dies.

As part of the effort to build support in Congress and in the states, the administration has begun to redefine the eligible population. Depending on one's point of view, it is using either sloppy or inaccurate estimates of the number of children who could receive the entitlement. For example, in a report entitled "Childhood Immunization Initiative: State Profiles," the Clinton administration estimates the number of eligible children from the ages of zero to five even though the emphasis of VFC was supposed to be on children of two and under. In any event, the administration's estimate of eligible children (aged zero to five) is, depending on which page you look at, either 36,286,804 or 37,241,971.[24] This is an impressive number considering there are only 22,000,000 children between the ages of zero and five in the entire country! In some state profiles, the number of eligible children exceeds the state's total population. As figure 6 shows, the administration estimates that there are 1,032,000 uninsured children in Vermont. This is amazing considering that only 576,000 people live in the entire state. The administration claims that this is a typographical error. It also managed to find exactly 1,032,000 eligibles in three other states: Pennsylvania, South Carolina, and Tennessee.

VFC Spending Rises Rapidly

The results of the ability to protect VFC as a children's entitlement are shown below. Figure 7 shows that between 1993 and 1995, immunization spending has increased from $349 million to almost $900 million, a rise of approximately 160 percent. As a result of its automatic and expansive character, VFC has become the fastest-growing entitlement in the past decade.

The growth of VFC cannot be controlled by Congress. While other entitlements have grown over the past thirty years, they have done so because Congress has decided to add new benefits or to expand eligibility. Apart from terminating the program, however, Congress has no control over the size and growth of VFC. Under the law, the only body that has control over VFC is an

FIGURE 6
Clinton Administration Estimate of
Vermont's Uninsured Children, Aged 0–5

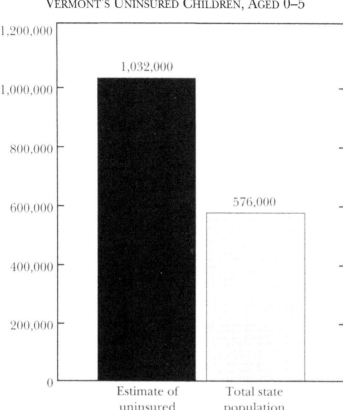

SOURCES: Department of Health and Human Services; Census Bureau.

informal, unelected body called the Advisory Committee on Immunization Practices (ACIP). ACIP advises CDCP about when vaccines should be administered and which ones should be used.

As a result, ACIP has become the appropriations committee for the VFC program. A recent ACIP meeting underscored the control the committee has over the size

FIGURE 7
PROJECTED INCREASES IN VFC SPENDING UNDER CLINTON PLAN, FY 1993–1997
(millions of dollars)

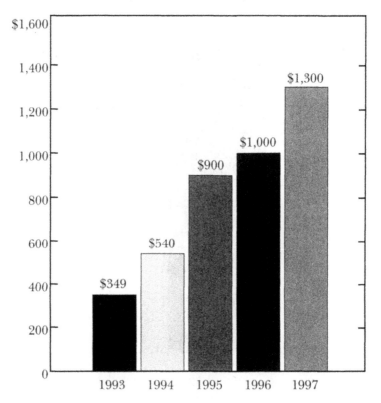

Source: U.S. Budget.

and content of the program. In this meeting, ACIP voted to expand coverage to include people up to age eighteen for existing vaccines and to add yet another.[25] This is in addition to the vaccines for hepatitis A and chicken pox that were added to the childhood immunization schedule in a previous meeting.

24

A recent article concerning ACIP's role in expanding the entitlement and the committee's free hand observes, "Depending on how its recommendations are interpreted, ACIP could effectively raise the number of doses to be purchased by tens of millions (for each new vaccine)."[26]

In 1995 alone, ACIP has added vaccines for influenza, a second measles shot for children eleven to twelve, and a hepatitis B shot for children eleven to twelve to the VFC entitlement. This expansion will add approximately $110 million to the VFC budget, bringing 1995's total to $990 million. Since ACIP has also recommended adding the newly approved hepatitis A and chicken pox shots, VFC spending could increase by another $300 million if the government buys more than what is required to immunize all two-year-olds.

VFC and the Perversion of Public Policy

The late Aaron Wildavsky observed that by using the rhetoric of crisis and failure to generate support for programs, public policy is perverted. To paraphrase Wildavsky, VFC was created by disparaging past progress and by convincing ourselves that we are not doing well and will soon be doing worse. The process of building up smaller dangers into larger ones "prevents us from setting priorities; because so many things are crises, without whose resolution it is alleged this nation cannot endure, everything must be done or nothing is worth doing."[27] In turn, the policy process is stymied because every problem requires extreme remedies. VFC was made possible by turning low immunization rates into a crisis. But in the process, VFC diverted and displaced resources that could have been used for other social purposes.

Relative to the larger primary health care needs of many poor children or the necessity for developing vaccines that prevent childhood diseases, low immunization rates represent a small problem medically and socially. Established as an entitlement that would wither away with the emergence of national health insurance, VFC is ensuring that substantial financial and political resources are being wasted over the fight to retain and expand the program—resources that could have been dedicated to other problems.

Low immunization rates can be overcome without VFC. We know that if parents are required to immunize their children or are reminded of its importance, children will get immunized at any age. Cost is no barrier to achieving higher immunization rates in localities where rates are low. The key is to link resources with parental responsibility and to provide states with flexibility to develop programs based on this principle. Accordingly, adding immunization funds to Medicaid block grants would allow states to apply money to any combination of activities deemed necessary. The CDCP and local health agencies could focus their time and talent on controlling disease and improving the public health in the pockets of greatest need. Companies could invest resources in a new generation of childhood vaccines.

The Clinton administration chose VFC as a symbol of its commitment to the goal of universal health care, and to the forces it would have to tame and control to achieve this victory. By elevating immunization rates into a national crisis, the White House was able to marshal substantial financial and political resources to enact an entitlement. As such, it will be extremely difficult to eliminate the program or halt its growth. In equal measure it will be difficult to invest in other, more worthy programs related to children's health. VFC is a failure not because of what it did not accomplish, but because of what it is doing to undermine other activities that improve the quality of immunization services in this country.

Notes

1. "Congress and the Nation," *Congressional Quarterly*, vol. V, Washington, D.C., 1982, p. 618.

2. Remarks by Donna Shalala, Secretary of Health and Human Services, Washington, D.C., April 1, 1993.

3. "Universal Immunization Initiative: Questions and Answers," Children's Defense Fund, February 8, 1993.

4. Joseph Tiang-Yau Liu and Sara Rosenbaum, "Medicaid and Childhood Immunizations: A National Study," Children's Defense Fund, Washington, D.C., January 1992, p. 1.

5. Shalala, Statement for the Joint Hearing of the Senate Committee on Labor and Human Resources and the House Energy and Commerce Committee Subcommittee on Health and the Environment, April 21, 1993.

6. Neither the administration's mishandling of the nation's vaccine supply nor the emergence of evidence that no immunization crisis exists, but rather immunization success, has stopped the program from growing. Instead, the fear of taking on a children's entitlement, even one with no real purpose, has insulated the program from any real criticism.

As is now fairly well known, the implementation of VFC has been plagued by delays in the effort to set up a distribution system and recruit physicians. Congress assumed that private vaccine companies would distribute government-supplied vaccines. But the price controls on vaccines left no margin for manufacturer delivery costs. As a result, the administration decided to set up its own distribution system. As part of its proposal, the administration was to have the General Services

Administration (GSA) handle shipping and storage out of a megawarehouse in New Jersey used for storing paint thinner and other odds and ends. Nearly 40 percent of the nation's pediatric vaccine supply was to be stored and handled by GSA, who in defending their ability to deliver vaccines pointed out that they successfully shipped frozen food to the Persian Gulf during Desert Storm. The warehouse idea was roundly criticized by the General Accounting Office and in the press. The proposal invited ridicule and was ultimately scrapped under pressure from Congress. In canceling it, the administration deflected attention from the larger and more important issue: whether VFC was actually necessary to begin with. Even though the GAO and others had noted that access to free vaccine was not a barrier to improving immunization rates, the value of the program never came under challenge. Not once did Congress or the press mount a sustained inquiry about whether centralized purchase and distribution of vaccine was efficient or worthwhile.

7. Walter Orenstein, M.D., Director, National Immunization Program, Centers for Disease Control and Prevention, U.S. Senate Subcommittee of the Committee of Appropriations, Washington, D.C., May 18, 1994, p. 21.

8. See note 5, supra. Note this exchange:

Senator Riegle: "The data I have been able to see...from CDC show that three-fourths of the two-year-olds who aren't fully immunized are in fact above poverty line. Is that right?"

Secretary Shalala: "Yes, Senator."

9. Statement at Albert Sabin Vaccine Foundation Conference on Private Insurance Coverage for Immunizations, Vista Hotel, Washington, D.C., February 20, 1995.

10. Elizabeth Weir, Sara Rosenbaum, et al., "Universal Distribution of Childhood Vaccines: The Experience of Twelve States," *Health Policy and Child Health*, vol. 2, Winter, 1994.

11. National Vaccine Advisory Committee, "The Measles Epidemic: The Problems, Barriers, and Recommendations," *Journal of the American Medical Association*, vol. 266, September 18, 1991, p. 1548.

12. Ibid.

13. Ibid., p. 1550.

14. Bernard Guyer, M.D., M.P.H.; Nancy Hughart, R.N., M.P.H.; et al., "Immunization Coverage and Its Relationship to Preventive Health Care Visits Among Inner-City Children in Baltimore," *Pediatrics*, vol. 94, July 1994, p. 57.

15. Ibid., pp. 56–57.

16. See Allan M. Arbeter, M.D., "A Study to Increase Immunization Coverage of Inner-City Minority Children in Philadelphia, Pennsylvania, Albert Einstein Medical Center, Philadelphia, July 2, 1993. Also, see David Wood, Cathy Sherbourne, et al., "Increasing Immunizations among Latino and African-American Preschool Children in Los Angeles," July 1993.

17. Tiang-Yau Liu and Rosenbaum, "Medicaid and Childhood Immunizations."

18. National Vaccine Advisory Committee, "The Measles Epidemic," p. 1550.

19. Statement of F.E. Thompson, Jr., M.D., M.P.H., State Health Officer, Mississippi State Department of Health, before the Committee on Finance of the United States Senate, May 4, 1995, p. 4.

20. Testimony of Dr. Orenstein.

21. What contributed to that success? Several factors. A general rise in social and economic status is positively related to an increase in health measures. In addition, for nearly twenty years, rich and poor alike have had equal access to adequate primary care. That is, in terms of having a medical home or a regular source of care, children of all income levels have strikingly similar levels of medical care, regardless of whether they are on Medicaid or private insurance, or whether they have insurance coverage or do not. According to the National Medical Expenditure Survey (NMES), fully 90 percent of all children under the age of one have a regular source of health care. Finally, the availability of antibiotics and vaccines for many infectious diseases has made disease prevention relatively easy and inexpensive to control.

Some analysts see a private doctor as a more constant source of care than other sources. Yet the NMES survey showed that most parents have a regular source of infant care. Eighty percent of black and 92 percent of white infants had a regular source of care. The poor were less likely to have a regular source compared with middle-class respondents (82 percent as opposed to 94 percent). Moreover, surveys show that children under the age of one from families in poverty visit a doctor for routine care (which NMES defines as visits for routine checkups and immunizations when nothing is wrong) at a slightly lower percentage. Eighty-seven percent of children under one year in poverty have visited a doctor for routine care, as compared with 97 percent of families with incomes above $40,000. The point is, immunization rates are much lower than the percentage of children who visited a doctor for routine care.

22. Weir, Rosenbaum, et al., "Universal Distribution of Childhood Vaccines."

23. Statement at Albert Sabin Vaccine Foundation Conference.

24. *Childhood Immunization Initiative: State Profiles*, U.S. Department of Health and Human Services, January 1995.

25. ACIP added influenza vaccine coverage for high-risk groups such as children with asthma; hepatitis B for high-risk groups under age eleven (instead of seven); and a dose for all children eleven to twelve not previously vaccinated with the hepatitis B vaccine. It also approved covering an additional group of children eighteen or under for a second dose of MMR.

26. Cheryl Pakolo Jones, "Should Vaccines outside Routine Ones Be Covered by VFC?" *Infectious Diseases in Children*, April 1994.

27. Aaron Wildavsky, "Dispelling America's Gloom: Why Bother?" *The American Enterprise*, vol. 1, March/April 1990, p. 26.

About the Author

ROBERT M. GOLDBERG is a senior research fellow at the Gordon Public Policy Center at Brandeis University and an associate director of the Center on Neuroscience, Behavior and Society at George Washington University. He has written extensively on health care policy and the effect of government regulation on biotechnology for such periodicals as the *Wall Street Journal,* the *Los Angeles Times,* and *Reader's Digest.*

Mr. Goldberg's research on the Vaccines for Children Program includes two Gordon Center reports: "Removing the Barriers," an analysis of the effect of VFC on immunization rates, and "Achieving the Promise," a study of how the VFC program will shape investment in vaccine research.

Mr. Goldberg received his Ph.D. in Public Policy from Brandeis University in 1984.

www.ingramcontent.com/pod-product-compliance
Lightning Source LLC
Jackson TN
JSHW011944131224
75386JS00041B/1559